Low Carb

Low Carb Diet Cookbook with Low Carb Keto Recipes for Batch Cooking

LELA GIBSON

CONTENTS

Introduction

I want to thank you and congratulate you for buying the book, *"Low Carb"*.

This book contains proven steps and strategies on how to prepare low carb keto recipes for batch cooking.

Low carb diets are continually gaining popularity due to their effectiveness in reversing type II diabetes, improving mental health and weight loss. However, it is one thing to know something is good for you and another thing to actually embrace it in your life.

While most people appreciate that a low carb diet is quite effective for weight loss, most people have a problem adopting such a diet owing to the time that one has to spend preparing and cooking your own meals.

Nevertheless, I have some good news for you. Thanks to batch cooking, you can adopt any kind of diet you want, including a low carb diet and not spend a lot of time cooking. You only need to spend some time preparing your meals in batches and once you are done, the only thing you need to do is just cook. How amazing is that?

If you want to learn more about batch cooking and some low carb recipes you can try out, this book has your back. You will learn how to prepare your meals in batches as well as low carb recipes that you can try out.

Thanks again for buying this book, I hope you enjoy it!

against the publisher for any reparation, damages, or monetary loss due to the information herein, either directly or indirectly.

Respective authors own all copyrights not held by the publisher.

The information herein is offered for informational purposes solely, and is universal as so. The presentation of the information is without contract or any type of guarantee assurance.

The trademarks that are used are without any consent, and the publication of the trademark is without permission or backing by the trademark owner. All trademarks and brands within this book are for clarifying purposes only and are the owned by the owners themselves, not affiliated with this document.

Low Carb Diet Broken Down

Before we look at batch cooking, let us try to understand a low carb diet or a keto diet. A low carb diet is simply a diet that restricts the amount of carbs eat in a day so that your body can tap into your fat stores and burn fat for energy. Most low carb diets limit your carbohydrate intake to 50-150 grams each day. Let us look at how much of the various macronutrients you can take while on a low carb diet:

Carbohydrates

Your carbohydrate intake as mentioned earlier should be 50-150 grams. This translates to around 20-25g net carbs in a day. This amount is important to ensure the body does not have access to enough carbs to burn for energy. Carbohydrates, which are broken down to glucose is your body's main or go-to source of energy. If you want your body to turn to burning fat for energy, you must limit your carbohydrates. If you do this, your body will have no other choice than to turn to another source of energy; it will burn fat.

Protein

20% of your calories should come from protein. Ensure you don't eat too much protein because of a process known as gluconeogenesis. In this process, the body converts excess protein to glucose and uses it to power its various functions. As you know by now, the body loves using glucose to meets its energy needs. This means you'll risk availing glucose for energy, if you take too much protein, which will not yield the results you are hoping for.

Fat

75% of your daily calorie intake should come from fat. Remember a low carb diet or the keto diet is based on fat burning. Your body will be relying on its stored fat and the fat you eat in order to power its functions. This is why fat should feature prominently whenever you sit down for a meal.

Why Batch Cooking

As you can imagine, in this era of fast foods, refined sugars and processed foods, it takes a bit of meal planning to ensure you meet the above macronutrient needs including keeping your carbohydrate intake low.

If you are quite busy and rarely have time to cook, you can easily get discouraged from following a low carb diet. This is because most foods that are readily available are usually quite high in carbohydrates. This is why you should figure out ways to make following this diet easier. One way you can simplify your life is by embracing batch cooking. This is where you make multiple recipes to eat throughout the week. Batch cooking has various benefits such as:

It is convenient

Batch cooking is convenient simply because it allows you some comfort you wouldn't have if you had to cook at least 3 meals each day. When you prepare your meals earlier, you will not have to deal with the rigorous process of cooking from scratch especially when you're tired or after a long day at work.

Saves time

Cooking every day especially if you have to prepare three meals or more involves a lot of work. Batch cooking lets you do all those little chores such as chopping, browning, shredding and baking at one go. Additionally, the preparation time and the cooking time does not change too much just because you're cooking in batches. In any case, adding a few more minutes to cook once a week is worth it if you will save more time during the week.

Makes cleaning easier

This is a huge plus as far as batch cooking is concerned. When preparing food, you need to use cutting boards, bowls, several pots, various spoons and even a food processor. After which when you are done preparing your meals, you have to wash these items. If you're cooking 3 times a day or even twice, you'll need to clean your cooking tools every time you cook. However, if you cook in batches, you'll lessen the cleaning work as you've already done the bulk of the work and cleaned the tools you used.

Enables you to meet your dietary needs

A major reason why you should embrace batch cooking is that it will help you meet your dietary needs. Think about it. The low carb diet requires planning. If you decide to eat certain foods at the spur of the moment, you will risk messing up. You must calculate your macros in order to ensure you don't overdo it when consuming carbohydrates. Batch cooking allows you to calculate your macros beforehand and freeze your meals in such a way that you'll be sure of the amounts you'll be eating. Your work would just be to select the meals that will help you meet your requirements for the day.

Also, batch cooking allows you to cook food for various family members and mark them. This way, it is much easier following a low carb diet even if other family members do not. You won't have to keep cooking two different meals every breakfast, lunch and dinner. You would just cook once and enjoy your meals throughout the week.

When batch cooking have the following things in mind:

Ensure there is headspace when freezing: Before freezing anything, enure that you wrap it well and you squeeze out any excess air. This will avoid freezer ban. In addition, ensure there is "headspace" especially when freezing soup because it normally expands.

Use muffin tins to get near perfect portions: If you don't want to store according to the servings, you can store in small portions in muffin tins. It is much easier and faster to reheat small portions. This will also ensure you don't waste food. Once the portions are set, pop them out and then bag them. You can reheat them any time you want.

When reheating already baked casseroles, simply put the

casserole in a cold oven and then preheating and cooking it for around 20 minutes. Ensure you don't put a frozen dish in a hot oven.

Select various recipes: Batch cooking is simply about cooking various meals to use for weeks to come. This means you can select four to five different recipes and set aside some time to prepare all of them. You should write your shopping list so that you can get all the ingredients ready. Ideally, you'd want to spend as little time as possible cooking.

Double up on recipes: There is no reason why you shouldn't double up in various recipes when you are batch cooking. Remember the keyword is batch. If a recipe only caters for 4 servings, you can double it up to make 8 servings.

Go easy on the vegetables: Vegetables tend to wilt when they are cooked. One thing you need to keep in mind is that eventually you will need to reheat the food when you want to eat it. When you reheat the vegetables, they may taste overcooked. This is why you should make a habit of only cooking vegetables slightly when you're batch cooking. Remove the vegetables from the heat at least 10 minutes before they are ready. This way, when you reheat them, they will be just right.

Make use of your food processor: Your food processor can help you out a lot when batch cooking. You can use it to blend onions or garlic or even vegetables such as carrots. This will make your work easier as it is no fun slicing many onions. You can use your food processor to slightly chop up various vegetables and add them to your soups or stews.

Let the food cool: Once you're done cooking, you should allow your food to sit for at least 30 minutes before placing it in your fridge for another 30 minutes. This will allow your food to cool down and then you can arrange it in the freezer. You should never leave food at room temperature for more than two hours before placing it in the freezer. If you do so, you'll allow bacteria to grow. Also, you should habitually defrost your food inside the refrigerator and not on counter tops.

Label the containers: It is easy to tell food apart when it is still in its uncooked state. However, this changes when the food is frozen and in containers. This is especially so when you cook in batches and have many containers that need to be identified. This is why you should carefully label the containers. Write down when you cooked the food and what is in the container. You can also include details such as the amount of carbs in the food. Remember to eat the food within three months to avoid losing its nutritional value and flavors.

Freeze in portions: When you freeze up food, it becomes one solid block. Thus, it makes little sense to freeze food without first dividing it into various portions. You need to determine how much food you'll need to eat for meals and divide the food accordingly. This way, you can easily remove the container you want and leave the rest in your freezer for later

Don't forget foods in the back: This is a point that needs to be emphasized. This is because once you get into the habit of batch cooking, you'll find yourself placing a lot of containers in the freezer and fridge. If you don't create a good system, you'll find yourself forgetting about some foods. Yes, it happens. Therefore, ensure that you rearrange your freezer at least once a month. This way, you can check to see if something had been placed in the back and forgotten. Also, make it a point to place the foods, which should be eaten first in front of the other containers.

In the following chapters, we will look at some low carb recipes that you can try out when batch cooking.

Breakfast

Breakfast Pizza

Servings: 8

Ingredients

1 cup cheese, shredded

2 cups peppers, sliced

8 oz sausage

1/4 teaspoon pepper

1/2 teaspoon salt

1/2 cup heavy cream

12 eggs

Directions

Preheat the oven to 350 degrees.

Microwave the peppers for 3 minutes and put aside.

Brown the sausage; you can do so in a cast iron skillet. Set it aside once it's done.

Mix together cream, eggs, salt and pepper and then place the mixture in the skillet. Cook for 5 minutes or until the sides set.

Place the mixture in the oven and bake for 20 minutes.

Remove from the oven, top up with peppers, sausage and cheese and then place it in the broiler for an additional 3 minutes.

Once done, let it sit for 5 minutes.

Serve and enjoy a slice. Freeze the remaining for later.

Nutritional information per serving: calories 307, fat 24.3g, protein 18.4g, carbs 2.6g, fiber 0.5g, net carbs 2.1g

Keto Breakfast Biscuits

Servings: 6

Ingredients

6 breakfast sausage patties, pre-cooked

2 ounces Colby Jack cheese, cubed

Pinch of salt and pepper

1 cup almond flour

2 eggs, beaten

2 cups mozzarella, shredded

2 ounces cream cheese

Directions

Preheat the oven to 400 degrees F.

Microwave the mozzarella and cream cheese for 30-second periods until the mozzarella starts melting; stir well to mix.

In a small bowl, mix the almond flour and the beaten egg and then add the cheese mixture and stir to combine. The dough may become a bit sticky. You can dust it with more flour before forming into a ball. Refrigerate the ball until the dough firms up.

Remove from the refrigerator and divide into 6 balls and then flatten each ball and place a sausage in the middle of each flattened dough. Add the cheese on top of each and then wrap the dough around. Do that for each portion.

Place the prepared dough into a muffin tin. Make sure you grease the tin first.

Bake for 12-15 minutes. The muffins should be golden and set. You can top up with additional mozzarella if you wish.

These biscuits freeze very well. If you wish to eat them, you need only to microwave for about one minute.

Nutritional information per serving: calories 250, fat 20g, protein 12g, net carbs 2g

Spinach and Feta Pie

Servings: 12

Ingredients

Grain-free piecrust

Salt and pepper to taste

1 tablespoon coconut flour

1 egg

150g almond meal

Spinach and Feta Filling

Salt and pepper to taste

Huge handful fresh mint, chopped

250g feta, crumbled

250g cream cheese, full fat

1/2 onion, finely diced

6 eggs, beaten

500g spinach, fresh or frozen

Directions

Use a fork to mix the ingredients for the crust.

Grease a 24cm pie dish or flan dish, line it with parchment paper and then pour the crust mixture onto it.

Take a piece of baking paper, place it on top of the mixture and then use a glass tumbler to flatten the crust.

Make holes in the crust using a fork to allow for an even bake.

Bake the crust for 15 minutes at 180C/350F. Remove and set aside.

Spinach and feta filling:

If you're using frozen spinach, defrost it and ensure you squeeze out the water to avoid ending up with a soggy pie.

Mix the spinach and the remaining ingredients ensuring that you leave some feta and cream cheese lumps.

Pour the mixture onto your piecrust and bake for 40 minutes at 180C/350F. The center should be cooked before you remove.

Refrigerate the leftovers for later. You can also refrigerate the pie after adding the filling and once ready to cook, use the above cooking directions.

Nutritional information per serving: calories 209, fat 16g, protein 10.6g, carbohydrates 4.2g, dietary fiber 2.2g, sugars 0.6g

Low Carb Breakfast Casserole

Servings: 9

Ingredients

1/4 teaspoon black pepper

1/4 teaspoon sea salt

2 tablespoons fresh parsley, chopped

2 cups cheddar cheese, divided

1/2 cup heavy cream

12 large eggs

6 cloves garlic, minced

1 lb. Breakfast sausage

Directions

Sauté the minced garlic in a greased skillet, for 1 minute or until it is fragrant.

Place the breakfast sausage in the skillet over medium-high heat and cook it for 10 minutes. Use a spatula to break it apart as it browns.

In the meantime, preheat your oven to 375F.

In a large bowl, mix the heavy cream, eggs, parsley, sea salt, black pepper and half of the cheddar cheese.

Grease the bottom of a casserole dish well and then arrange the crumbled sausage at the bottom. Spread it evenly. If you want to use any pre-cooked vegetables, add them at this stage.

Spread the egg mixture evenly over the sausage and top up with the remaining cheddar cheese.

Bake for about 30 minutes until the cheese melts and the eggs are set. Remove and freeze appropriately.

Nutritional information per serving: calories 281, fat 23g, protein 17g, carbohydrates 1g, dietary fiber 0.1g, sugars 0g

Lunch

Eggplant Moussaka

Servings: 10

Ingredients

300 grams thick cream

112 grams cheddar cheese

20 grams Italian herb

410 grams ardmona chopped tomatoes mixed herbs

1 carrot, diced

1 red onion, diced

1 eggplant/aubergine

3 cloves garlic

1 kg beef mince, Grass-fed

Splenda to taste.125 grand Philadelphia cream cheese

Directions

Thinly slice the eggplant, fry it in coconut oil and then set it aside.

In a pan, sauté the red onion, carrot and garlic and then add the mince meat and brown it. Add the ardmona, Italian herb mix, tomatoes and then season with salt and splenda and remove from heat.

Prepare the cheese cream sauce by frying thin slices of cream cheese together with 300g of thick cream. Make sure you add the cream bit by bit and then add splenda to taste. Set aside.

Spread a layer of eggplant in a casserole dish, then the meat mixture and then add a layer of cheese sauce and a layer of meat sauce and finally a layer of shredded cheddar. If you're cooking in bigger batches, start with a layer of eggplant and then meat and finally cheese sauce and repeat.

Bake for 15 minutes at 180 degrees/ 350F.

Serve and enjoy. You can freeze leftovers for later.

Nutritional information per serving: fat 30g, protein 24g, carbs 9g

Portobello Pesto Pizza

Servings: 4

Ingredients

For the Portobello pesto pizza:

4 ounces grated mozzarella

11/2 tablespoons olive oil

2 medium tomatoes, sliced

4 Portobello mushrooms

For the basil pesto:

3 tablespoons olive oil

1/2 small avocado

1 garlic clove, peeled

2 cups loosely packed basil leaves

2 tablespoons of pine nuts or walnuts

Directions

Preheat the oven to 400 degrees F.

In a food processor, prepare the basil pesto by pulsing together the pine nuts, avocado, garlic and basil. Add olive oil and pulse some more to get a sauce-like consistency. Season the basil pesto with salt and pepper.

Remove the stems from the mushrooms and scrape out the inside gills using a spoon. Use olive oil to brush both sides of the mushrooms.

Place the mushrooms on a sheet own with the caps side down. Place 1/3 of the pesto onto the mushrooms, then spread tomatoes, and cheese on top.

Bake for 15-18 minutes or until the cheese is bubbly. Enjoy and freeze the leftovers.

Nutritional information per serving: calories 303, fat 29g, carbs 10g, dietary fiber 4g, sugar 1g, protein 13g

Mushroom Cauliflower Burgers

Servings: 6

Ingredients

Salt and pepper to taste

6+ tablespoons almond flour

1/2 teaspoon dried rosemary

1/2 head of cauliflower, grated (or 2cups cauliflower)

8 oz mushrooms, chopped into small pieces

1 tablespoon olive oil

1 clove garlic, minced

1/2 yellow onion, chopped

Toppings: ketchup, spinach, mustard tahini

Directions

Combine all the toppings ingredients in a small bowl, and set aside.

In a flat pan or cast iron skillet, add the olive oil and cook the onion over medium heat for 2 minutes.

Add the garlic and mushrooms and then sprinkle the dried rosemary on top. Stir with a wooden spoon and cook for an additional 3-4 minutes or until the mushrooms are soft.

Add the cauliflower rice and stir for 1 more minute; season with salt and pepper. Remove from heat and let it cool down to room temperature.

In the meantime, preheat your oven to 400 degrees F and then line the baking sheet with parchment paper.

Once you can handle the cauliflower mixture comfortably, add 2 tablespoons of almond flour at a time and mix everything. Once mixed, form 6 burger patties. The patties should stick together. You can add more flour if you notice they are cracking too much. Place the patties on the prepared baking sheet.

Bake for 30 minutes at 400 degrees F or until the patties are golden brown on top. You can broil for a few last minutes if you wish.

When you're ready to eat, you can serve with spinach, tomatoes, buns, lettuce, red onion and pickles if you wish. Otherwise, freeze for later.

Nutritional information per serving: calories 83, total fat 6g, total carbs 5.5g, dietary fiber 2g, sugars 2.1g, protein 3.6g

Keto Cabbage Lasagna

Servings: 20

Ingredients

1/4 cup Parmesan, grated (optional)

32 ounces fresh mozzarella cheese, sliced or shredded

40 ounces marinara sauce with no added sugar

2 pounds ground meat, browned

3 large eggs

1/4 cup dried parsley, optional

11/2 cups Parmesan cheese, grated

3 lbs. ricotta cheese

1 head cabbage

Directions

Carefully separate the cabbage leaves and parboil for 5-10 minutes in salted boiling water. Once done, use a towel to drain excess water.

In a bowl, mix Parmesan cheese, ricotta, eggs and parsley and then set aside.

Add marinara sauce to the browned meat and stir.

Pour 3/4 cup of the in the baking pan. You can use an 11 by 15-inch pan.

Spread a layer of the cooked cabbage leaves over the sauce in the baking pan.

Place half the ricotta cheese mixture on top of the cabbage leaves.

Add the remaining sauce and then spread half the mozzarella cheese on top.

Repeat the layers and then top up with any additional Parmesan cheese if you wish.

Bake for about 25 minutes at 350F.

Nutritional information per serving: calories 451, carbs 9g, dietary fiber 1g, sugars 3g, protein 27g

Dinner

Quinoa Burgers

Servings: 6

Ingredients

For the tomato olive topping:

1 teaspoon red wine vinegar or lemon juice

1 tablespoon chopped fresh basil

1 tablespoon chopped fresh parsley

1/4 cup pitted kalamata olives, diced

1 cup cherry tomatoes, quartered

For the burgers:

Lettuce for serving

Olive oil, for cooking the burgers

1 tablespoon finely chopped fresh basil

1 tablespoon minced fresh parsley

1/4 cup crumbled feta cheese, plus additional for serving

1 large egg

1/4 teaspoon ground black pepper

1/2 teaspoon dried oregano

1/2 teaspoon kosher salt

1 cup old fashioned rolled oats

1 (15-ounce) can chickpeas, rinsed and drained

2 cloves garlic, minced

1/4 cup chopped sundried tomatoes (not olive oil packed)

1/2 cup uncooked quinoa, millet, farro or similar grain

Directions

Add the quinoa and 1 cup of water into a saucepan, and bring to a boil. Lower the heat to a simmer, cover and cook for 15 minutes. Remove the quinoa from the heat and allow it to stand for 5 minutes. Uncover the pan and use a fork to fluff the quinoa and then set it aside.

In the meantime, put the sundried tomatoes in a bowl, cover them with very hot water and let it stand for 5 minutes in order to rehydrate. Drain and set aside.

In a food processor, blend quinoa, oats, chickpeas, oregano, garlic, salt and pepper. Add the egg and continue to pulse to combine.

Transfer the mixture to a mixing bowl and then add the feta, basil, sundried tomatoes and parsley and form 6 patties.

Freeze the patties in the refrigerator until you're ready to cook them.

To cook them, add olive oil to a large skillet and brown the patties for 4 minutes on each side.

In a small bowl, mix the toppings ingredients. Serve the burgers with lettuce, tomato olive oil mixture and your toppings.

Nutritional information per serving: calories 389, fat 7.2g, carbs 67.5g, fiber 12g, sugar 5.3g, protein 26.6g

Bacon Turkey Burgers

Servings: 8-10

Ingredients

1/2 teaspoon pepper

1 teaspoon salt

3 cloves garlic

1/2 medium onion

2 medium zucchini

1/2 lb bacon

2 1/2 lbs ground turkey

Directions

Preheat the oven to 350 degrees F.

Slice the bacon and cook over medium heat. The bacon should be crispy. Remove and drain on paper towels. Once the bacon is cool, chop it finely.

Set aside 1 tablespoon of the bacon fat. Use a food processor or grater to shred the zucchini. Finely chop the garlic and the onion.

Heat the bacon fat in a skillet over medium heat and sauté

the onion and garlic.

In a large bowl, mix all the ingredients and then form the mixture into 8-10 patties.

In a large skillet, brown the patties for 3 minutes per side. Remove and place them on a baking sheet lined using parchment paper.

Bake for 15 minutes or until cooked through.

Serve with lettuce. You can freeze the patties for later.

Nutritional information per serving: calories 354, fat 22g, carbs 2.5g, fiber 1g, sugar 1g, protein 40g

Spicy, Smoky Sweet Chili

Servings: 6

Ingredients

1/4 teaspoon cayenne pepper or to taste

1/2 teaspoon cumin

1/2 teaspoon onion powder

1/2 teaspoon garlic powder

3/4 teaspoon salt

1 teaspoon smoked paprika

3 tablespoons chili powder

15oz can black beans, drained and rinsed

15oz can baked beans

29oz can tomato sauce

Salt and pepper

2 garlic cloves, minced

1 large shallot or 1 small onion, chopped

1 lb ground beef

Toppings: sour cream, chopped green onions, shredded

cheddar cheese

Directions

Brown the ground beef, garlic, onion and shallot in a large skillet, over medium heat and then season with salt and pepper.

Add the other ingredients and simmer for 30 minutes. Remember to stir once or twice.

Place the ground beef into a 5-6 quart crock pot and then add the remaining ingredients and stir.

Close the lid and cook for 4-6 hours on low. Freeze in individual portions.

Nutritional information per serving: calories 354, fat 6g, carbs 42.9g, fiber 11.1g, sugar 14g, protein 33.6g

Snacks

Peanut Butter Chia Granola Bars

Servings: 12

Ingredients

1/4 teaspoon kosher salt

1 teaspoon cinnamon

1 teaspoon vanilla extract

1/3 cup honey

2/3 cup creamy peanut butter (refrain from using the kind that needs refrigeration)

1/4 cup chia seeds

1/4 cup uncooked millet or uncooked quinoa

1/2 cup roughly chopped nuts of your choice

11/3 cups old fashioned rolled nuts

1/2 cup desired mix-ins: chopped dried dates, chopped dried apricots, raisins, dried cherries, chocolate chips, etc

Directions

Optional - Preheat the oven to 350 degrees F. In an ungreased baking sheet, place the oats, quinoa or millet, nuts and chia seeds and bake for about 10 minutes or until lightly golden. Remove and set aside.

Line a baking dish with parchment paper or plastic wrap, lightly spray with cooking spray and then set aside.

In a saucepan over medium-low heat, add the honey and peanut butter and stir until creamy and smooth. Remove the mixture from the heat and then add cinnamon, vanilla and salt and stir to combine.

In a large bowl, mix the millet or quinoa, oats, nuts and chia seed. Spread the peanut butter mixture on top and stir using a rubber spatula to coat the ingredients. If you intend to use chocolate, allow the mixture to cool for 1-2 minutes before stirring any other mix-ins.

Spread the mixture on the baking sheet and use the spatula to press down firmly to ensure the mixture is spread tightly and evenly.

Refrigerate for 2 hours and then slice into bars. You can freeze the bars for later

Nutritional information per serving: calories 218, fat 11.5g, carbs 25.5g, fiber 3g, sugar 13g, protein 7g

Cocoa Butter Fat Bombs

Servings: 12

Ingredients

1 teaspoon sea salt

1 scant teaspoon stevia extract or 1/4 cup swerve

2 tablespoons ground golden flax seeds

4 oz cocoa butter

1/2 cup grass-fed butter or coconut oil

1/2 cup almond butter or unsweetened peanut butter

Directions

In a saucepan over medium-high heat, proceed heat several cups of water and then put a pyrex bowl on top of it.

Add all the ingredients into the bowl, melt and mix. Gently pour the mixture into silicone molds. Alternatively, you can pour it into lined mini muffin tins.

Freeze the mixture for at least 1 hour before serving. You can store the fat bombs in the refrigerator for 1-2 weeks.

Nutritional information per serving: calories 96, protein 4g, fat 10.5g, total carbs 3g, fiber 1g, net carbs 2g

Sun-Dried Tomato and Feta Meatballs

Servings: 16

Ingredients

2 tablespoons water

1/4 cup almond flour

1/2 teaspoon garlic powder

1 egg

1 tablespoon thyme leaves (or 1/2 teaspoon dried thyme)

2 tablespoons (.5 oz) sundried tomatoes, chopped

1/4 cup crumbled feta cheese

1 lb ground turkey

Olive oil for frying

Directions

Mix all the ingredients except the olive oil and then divide into 16 meatballs.

In a large sauté pan, add the olive oil and fry the meatballs. The meatballs should be browned and crisp. You can fry for 3-4 minutes before turning over and frying for an additional 3-4 minutes.

Remove the meatballs and place them on paper towels.

Serve and enjoy. You can serve with spaghetti squash and marinara sauce for a complete meal. These meatballs freeze well.

Nutritional information per serving: calories 89, fat 8g, net carbs 0.65g, protein 6g

Green Smoothie

Servings: 5

Ingredients

2 cups mixed berries

1 ½ cups unsweetened coconut milk

4 cups unsweetened coconut water

¼ cup chia seeds

½ cup unsweetened shredded coconut

½ cup protein powder

8 cups spinach

Directions

Put the ingredients in the blender starting with the pineapple, then spinach, protein powder, followed by coconut, the chia seeds and finally almond milk and coconut water. You may need to make the smoothie in 2-3 batches.

Blend until you achieve a smooth consistency. Taste and adjust the sweetness, then blend again.

Pour the smoothie into 5 mason jars making sure that you leave a little headspace, put the lid and pop into the freezer.

To thaw, it is best to leave the smoothie at room temperature for a few hours or overnight in the fridge.

Nutritional information per serving: calories 220.4, Protein 28g, Fat 9.6g, Net carbs 5.8g

I need your help...

Thank you again for buying this book!

As you have learned, it is possible to simplify your lifestyle and enjoy healthy meals. You can do this by embracing batch cooking. Batch cooking gives you the freedom to enjoy various low carb meals throughout the week without spending a lot of time in the kitchen. You just need to make your meal plan, get your ingredients ready and get cooking.

Finally, if you enjoyed this book, would you be kind enough to leave a review for this book on Amazon?

I want to reach as many people as I can with this book, and more reviews will help me accomplish that!

Bonus: Subscribe To The Free Weight Loss Report

When you subscribe to Freedom Destination via email, you will get free access to an ebook. All you have to do is enter your email address to get instant access.

The Introduction Manual is more than just an introduction to the diet. Instead, it discusses the science behind how we gain and lose weight as well as what absolutely needs to be done to attack that stubborn body fat that, until now, has been so challenging to get rid of.

Here are the preview of what you'll get:

- Rapid Weight Loss
- How This System Works
- Why This Diet
- Why 3 Weeks?
- 21 Days To Make A Habit
- Fat Loss VS. Weight Loss
- Nutrients

- Protein, Fat, Carbohydrates

- The Food Pyramid And Obesity

- Fiber

- Metabolism

- How We Get Fat

- Triglycerides

- How To Get Thin

- Diet Overview

- Meal Frequency

- Water

- Diet Essentials

- Let's Get Started

You can access it here: http://bit.ly/2tUb9cp

www.ingramcontent.com/pod-product-compliance
Lightning Source LLC
Chambersburg PA
CBHW070053260726
48658CB00002B/870